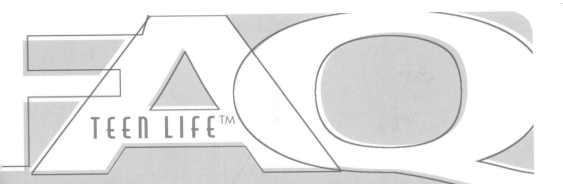

TEEN LIFE™

FREQUENTLY ASKED QUESTIONS ABOUT

Concussions

Linda
Bickerstaff

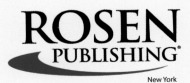

ROSEN
PUBLISHING®

New York

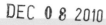

Published in 2010 by The Rosen Publishing Group, Inc.
29 East 21st Street, New York, NY 10010

Copyright © 2010 by The Rosen Publishing Group, Inc.

First Edition

Library of Congress Cataloging-in-Publication Data

Bickerstaff, Linda.
Frequently asked questions about concussions / Linda Bickerstaff.—1st ed.
    p. cm.—(FAQ: teen life)
Includes index.
ISBN 978-1-4358-3513-9 (library binding)
1. Brain Popular works.—Concussion I. Title.
RC394.C7B53 2010
612.8'2—dc22

                                            2009016319

Manufactured in Malaysia

CPSIA Compliance Information: Batch #TWW10YA: For Further Information contact Rosen Publishing, New York, New York at 1-800-237-9932

Contents

Chapter one

WHAT IS A CONCUSSION?

Have you ever hit your head really hard—hard enough to "see stars" and get a headache? If you have, you may have experienced a concussion. A concussion is a mild brain injury usually caused by a bump or blow to the head. Concussions can occur even if you aren't hit directly on the head. Any blow to your body that causes your head to violently snap around can cause your brain to hit the inside of your skull. The result will probably be a concussion. Concussions are also called mild traumatic brain injuries (MTBIs).

It is thought that as many as four thousand people get concussions every day in the United States. The actual number is probably a lot higher. For young children and adults, most concussions occur as the result of falls or automobile accidents. Accidents and falls associated with bicycling and other recreational activities, such as skating and skateboarding, are common

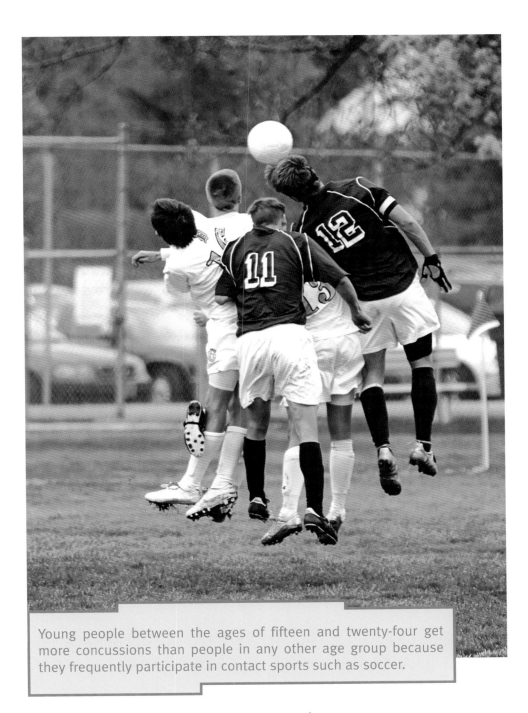

Young people between the ages of fifteen and twenty-four get more concussions than people in any other age group because they frequently participate in contact sports such as soccer.

causes of concussions in older children. Young people between the ages of fifteen and twenty-four have more concussions than those in any other age group. The reason for this is because most of them drive cars, ride bicycles, and play sports. These are the three activities most commonly associated with brain injuries.

Brain Basics

Your brain may weigh as much as 3 pounds (1 kilogram). It's about as thick and firm as a scoop of ice cream. It is protected by your skull and by a clear, colorless liquid called cerebral spinal fluid (CSF). The CSF surrounds the brain and acts as a shock absorber to keep it from hitting your skull every time you move your head. It also brings some nutrients to the brain and carries away some of the waste materials made by the brain.

The largest part of your brain is the cerebrum. It sits just beneath the skull and takes up much of the space within the skull. The cerebrum is divided into two halves by a deep groove called a sulcus. Each half is called a cerebral hemisphere. The right cerebral hemisphere controls the functions of the left side of the body, and the left cerebral hemisphere controls the right side of the body. The two halves communicate by a thick bundle of nerves in the front of the brain called the corpus callosum. These nerves carry messages back and forth between the two hemispheres.

Shallower grooves divide each hemisphere into four parts called lobes. These lobes are the frontal, temporal, parietal, and occipital lobes. The frontal lobes sit just behind your eyes. They

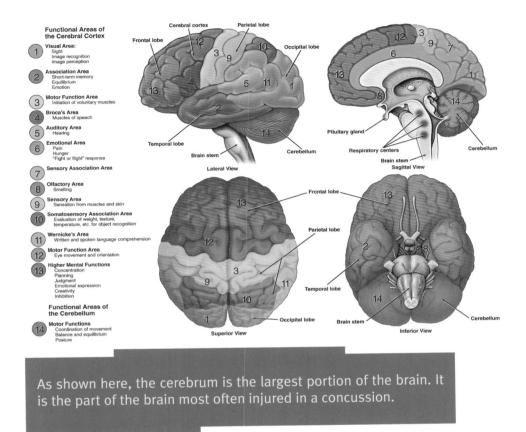

Functional Areas of the Cerebral Cortex

1. **Visual Area:**
   Sight
   Image recognition
   Image perception

2. **Association Area**
   Short-term memory
   Equilibrium
   Emotion

3. **Motor Function Area**
   Initiation of voluntary muscles

4. **Broca's Area**
   Muscles of speech

5. **Auditory Area**
   Hearing

6. **Emotional Area**
   Pain
   Hunger
   "Fight or flight" response

7. **Sensory Association Area**

8. **Olfactory Area**
   Smelling

9. **Sensory Area**
   Sensation from muscles and skin

10. **Somatosensory Association Area**
    Evaluation of weight, texture,
    temperature, etc. for object recognition

11. **Wernicke's Area**
    Written and spoken language comprehension

12. **Motor Function Area**
    Eye movement and orientation

13. **Higher Mental Functions**
    Concentration
    Planning
    Judgment
    Emotional expression
    Creativity
    Inhibition

Functional Areas of the Cerebellum

14. **Motor Functions**
    Coordination of movement
    Balance and equilibrium
    Posture

Cerebral cortex · Parietal lobe · Frontal lobe · Occipital lobe · Temporal lobe · Brain stem · Cerebellum · Pituitary gland · Respiratory centers · Lateral View · Sagittal View · Superior View · Inferior View

As shown here, the cerebrum is the largest portion of the brain. It is the part of the brain most often injured in a concussion.

control your ability to think and solve problems. They also determine how long you can concentrate on something. They control your emotions—whether you become angry, sad, or happy. Your personality and ability to interact with other people are also controlled by the frontal lobes.

The temporal lobes are located near your ears and are involved with hearing. They make it possible for you to understand words that are spoken to you. They're also responsible for

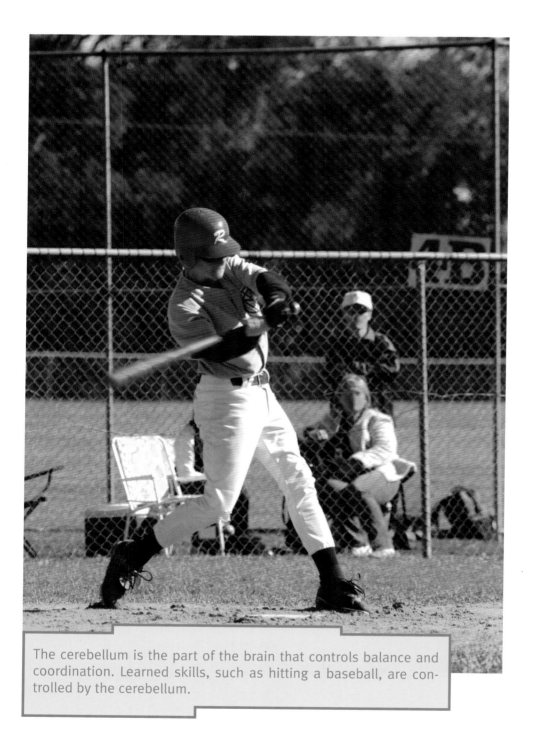

The cerebellum is the part of the brain that controls balance and coordination. Learned skills, such as hitting a baseball, are controlled by the cerebellum.

how well you remember events that happened a long time ago (long-term memory), as well as those things that just happened yesterday (short-term memory).

The parietal lobes are located on top of the cerebrum and behind the frontal lobes. They are involved with interpreting information gathered by the five senses: sight, hearing, smell, taste, and touch. For example, your parietal lobes help you tell the difference between the smell of freshly baked cookies and the smell of your unwashed gym socks. The parietal lobes are also the areas of the brain that control your ability to solve problems using numbers, write words, and draw pictures. These lobes also communicate with the temporal lobes to coordinate speech and understanding.

The last lobes of the cerebral hemispheres are the occipital lobes. They are found at the back of the brain and control most of the brain's vision function. These parts of the brain help you interpret what your eyes see. If these lobes are injured, you may not be able to tell the difference between colors, shapes, or words. People who are hit on the back of the head may see bright lights or "stars" and even think they see things that aren't really there.

Located under the occipital lobes of the cerebrum is the cerebellum, the second major part of the brain. The cerebellum controls balance and coordination. It also controls skills that you've likely learned to do, such as swinging a baseball bat or riding a bicycle. If this part of the brain is injured, you may have to relearn activities that you easily did before you were injured.

The third major part of the brain is located at the bottom of the brain just above the spinal cord. This is the brain stem. The

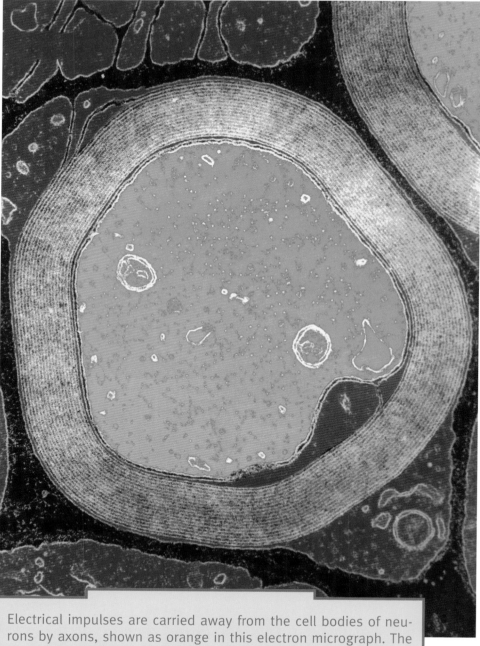

Electrical impulses are carried away from the cell bodies of neurons by axons, shown as orange in this electron micrograph. The axon's insulating myelin sheath is shown in green.

brain stem acts sort of like a switchboard, regulating the flow of information between the brain and the rest of your body. It controls all basic body functions like breathing, swallowing, heart rate, and blood pressure, as well as doing many other things.

If you look at a piece of the cerebrum (or cerebellum) under a microscope, you will see that it's made up of millions of nerve cells called neurons. The bodies of these cells, where all the work is done, are found in a thin outer layer of the cerebrum called the cerebral cortex. Projecting off of the cell bodies are axons, which are long, stringlike structures that make up the "wiring system" of the brain. Axons carry messages in the form of electrical impulses or charges from the cell bodies to other parts of the brain. Like electrical wires that are covered with a plastic coating, axons are covered with a special coating of fat called myelin. This layer is important because it keeps the electrical impulses that are being carried down the axons from being lost or "shorted out," and it may actually speed up their transmission.

What Happens to the Brain in a Concussion?

Concussions do not cause structural damage to the brain that can be seen on X-rays or scans of the brain. Instead, concussions cause injuries to brain cells and affect how they function. Normal neurons will not "fire" or send out electrical impulses unless they are stimulated by chemicals called excitatory neurotransmitters. When a concussion occurs, excessive amounts of these neurotransmitters are released in a widespread area of the brain around the site of the injury. The neurons are overstimulated or excited, and they begin to send out large numbers of irregular electrical impulses that can't be transmitted by axons to the rest of the brain. As a result, some brain functions are slowed down or stop completely until the neurons heal. Sometimes, the axons themselves are injured in a concussion. They may be stretched or their insulating myelin sheaths may be broken so that they can't transmit electrical currents normally.

How Will I Know If I Have a Concussion?

If you receive a blow to your head that causes a concussion, how will you feel? How are you likely to act? You may see bright lights, get a headache, feel dizzy, or have other feelings that are not normal for you. These feelings are called symptoms. These are effects you actually experience. Your teammates, coaches, athletic trainers, and team doctor may notice that you seem confused or "not all there." They may see you stagger when you try to walk. The ways you look and act can be signs of a concussion. No two people who have concussions will have the exact same signs and symptoms. Signs and symptoms help doctors determine if you've had a concussion. The disappearance of these effects helps doctors and coaches know how well your brain is healing.

Physical Signs and Symptoms of Concussions

Having pain in your head is the most common physical symptom of a concussion. About 85 percent of people who have concussions have headaches. Sometimes, this symptom persists for months. Another symptom of a concussion is dizziness. You may feel as if you are spinning around or that the things around you are spinning. You may also feel nauseated, or sick to your stomach, and may throw up. When you try to stand up or walk, you may be unsteady. Some people with concussions may see bright lights or two images instead of one when they look at something. Bright lights and loud noises make their headaches more severe. About 10 percent of people who experience concussions will lose consciousness, or get "knocked out." Others may pass out and have uncontrolled jerking of their arms and legs. This condition is called a seizure.

Physical signs of concussions include moving clumsily or staggering. You may have a vacant look on your face as if you are not "all there," or your speech may be difficult to understand. Unusual movements, seizures, sleepiness or unconsciousness, and vomiting are not only symptoms of concussions that a person experiences, but they are also signs that trainers, coaches, and doctors look for.

Cognitive Signs and Symptoms of Concussions

We use the word "cognitive" when referring to brain functions associated with thinking, learning, remembering, problem solving, and understanding, among others. Signs and symptoms of cognitive impairment include disorientation, or not knowing where you are or what is going on. You may also have trouble focusing your attention on something. For instance, if someone asks you a question, you may be unable to think about the question long enough to come up with an answer. You may also be unable to remember what happened after experiencing the concussion. This is called post-traumatic amnesia. People who experience concussions are almost always confused. They don't seem to be able to figure out what is going on. They repeatedly ask the same questions but are unable to understand the answers that they are given.

Coaches frequently ask teachers to report any student athlete who suddenly begins doing poorly on tests or who seems to have

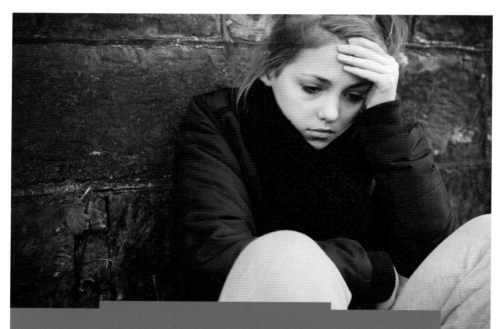

Emotional problems such as depression, as seen in this teen, may be signs and symptoms of an unrecognized concussion.

trouble learning. They know that playing sports can take time away from schoolwork and lead to slipping grades, but they also know that a concussion can make it difficult for a student to learn. Poor academic performance in a student athlete may be a sign of an unrecognized or an incompletely resolved concussion.

Emotional or Behavioral Signs and Symptoms of Concussions

Generally, emotional and behavioral signs and symptoms of concussions don't occur immediately. Sometimes, however, they are the first signs that something "just isn't right." Concussion victims who are usually pleasant and easygoing may become cranky and hard to get along with. They may lose interest in activities that they ordinarily enjoy. Crying, feeling very sad, being especially unkind to others, or being easily angered may be signs and symptoms of an unrecognized concussion.

two

HOW WILL MY DOCTOR DECIDE IF I HAVE HAD A CONCUSSION?

Most doctors have a routine they follow every time they see you. They take a history from you to find out what happened and what your symptoms are. They examine you to see if you have any signs that will help them decide what is going on. They then "make a diagnosis" or decide what they think the problem is. Most of the time, they order laboratory tests or X-rays to confirm their diagnosis. In the case of concussions, however, there aren't any laboratory tests or readily available X-rays that give information about your brain. The neurons that have been injured are simply too small to be imaged, even with powerful computed tomography (CT) scans and magnetic resonance imaging (MRI) scans. Some concussion victims who are seen in emergency rooms do have CT scans, however.

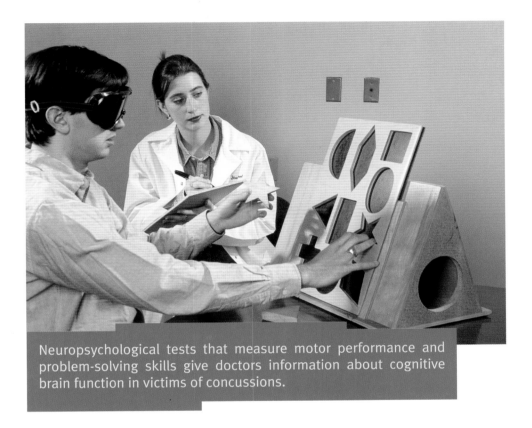

Neuropsychological tests that measure motor performance and problem-solving skills give doctors information about cognitive brain function in victims of concussions.

These are done to make sure they have no evidence of a more serious brain injury. But CT scans don't help make the diagnosis of a concussion.

Tests of Brain Function

Although your doctor has no readily available ways to "look" at the injured neurons in your brain after you have a concussion, he or she can do studies to determine how well your brain is working. The studies the doctor uses are neuropsychological tests. They can be used not only to help your doctor make the diagnosis of a concussion but also to help determine how fast your brain can heal itself. These tests measure how well you can think, whether or not you can perform simple math problems, how well you can concentrate, how well you can remember, and several other skills. These are all tests of cognitive function. They also test how quickly you can do something after being told to do it. This is called your reaction time and is one way of measuring coordination.

The physical symptoms that you have with your concussion may disappear quickly, but cognitive symptoms can last longer. In the past, people who experienced concussions were given a standardized group of neuropsychological tests shortly after they experienced their concussions. If the tests showed abnormalities, they were repeated every few days until all tests were normal. This was an indication that the brain was healed. These tests took several hours, required a lot of skill on the part of the person giving them, and took a long time to interpret. Fortunately, newer technology has led to the development of computerized neurocognitive testing. Programs that use this technology give precise information about a person's brain function. They're also faster, easier to administer and take, and are much less expensive than standard neuropsychological tests.

Two of the latest programs to be developed for neurocognitive testing are central nervous system vital signs (CNS VS) and immediate post-concussion assessment and cognitive testing

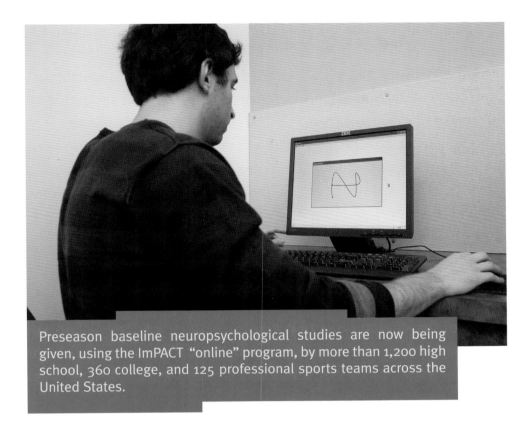

Preseason baseline neuropsychological studies are now being given, using the ImPACT "online" program, by more than 1,200 high school, 360 college, and 125 professional sports teams across the United States.

(ImPACT). These tests are given "online" using computer software programs. They are partially interpreted by computer, but they also require interpretation by physicians or psychologists who are trained in the programs. Doctors get the most information from these studies if the person taking them has had a baseline test with which to compare them. Athletes competing in sports where concussions commonly occur may have neurocognitive testing as part of their preseason physical evaluations. These serve as baseline studies that can be used to compare with studies taken if they experience concussions during the year. More than 1,200 high schools, 360 colleges and universities, and 125 professional sports teams nationwide now use ImPACT for preseason baseline studies and for testing if an athlete experiences a concussion during the sports season.

CNS VS and ImPACT are also used in sports medicine clinics and emergency rooms to evaluate neurocognitive function in patients displaying signs and symptoms of concussions. Psychologists and others who follow patients who've had concussions use these tests to help determine when brain healing occurs.

Screening Tests for Concussions

Many of the concussions that young people experience happen while they are playing on sports teams. It's important for coaches, athletic trainers, and team physicians to evaluate them immediately wherever the injuries occur. Tests that can be done quickly on the sidelines of a playing field are called screening tests. These short tests of neurocognitive function indicate whether or not an athlete has had a concussion.

There are several standardized tests that trainers and team physicians use for screening purposes. Many coaches and athletic trainers carry cards in their pockets that have neurocognitive test questions printed on them. If you are injured, they pull out the cards and ask you the questions, which might include: "Where is the game being played?," "What position do you play on the team?," or "What quarter or period is the game in?" These questions test your orientation—who you are, where you are, and what time it is. The trainer will then ask you to do some easy tests to check your ability to concentrate and solve problems. These might include having you repeat the order of the months backward or subtract numbers backward. The trainer also wants to know if you have amnesia, so he or she will ask questions to see if you remember the events that happened before you were hit.

Included in the screening tests are ones designed to test your balance and coordination. One test the trainer may do is have you stand in various positions with your eyes closed to see if you have to change your position or open your eyes to keep from falling over. Trainers and team doctors use the information from these tests to decide the next step in your evaluation and care. They and your coach also use them to decide whether or not you can return to play.

What's New in Neurocognitive Screening?

Two new high-tech methods of neurocognitive screening have been developed and are presently undergoing clinical trials. DETECT, which stands for "display enhanced testing for cognitive impairment and traumatic brain injury," is a device that can be used anywhere as a screening tool for concussions. It includes a virtual reality (VR) headset that covers an athlete's eyes, a set of earphones, and a video game controller. Groups of words or figures of different shapes and colors appear in the VR display. The player receives commands through the earphones

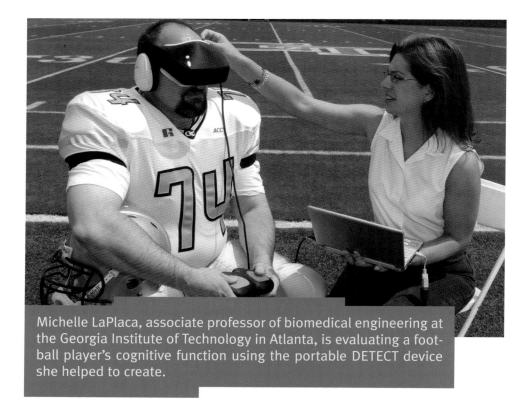

Michelle LaPlaca, associate professor of biomedical engineering at the Georgia Institute of Technology in Atlanta, is evaluating a football player's cognitive function using the portable DETECT device she helped to create.

and pushes buttons on the controller to do what he or she is told to do. The device measures how quickly the athlete can do the tasks (reaction time) and whether the athlete's answers are right or wrong. A computer interprets the data so that trainers and team doctors have almost immediate information about the athlete's cognitive function. The athlete's reaction time measures his or her coordination. The entire set of tests can be completed in about seven minutes. One of the most important features of DETECT is its portability. It can not only be used on the sidelines at sporting events but also can be used in emergency rooms, clinics, and even on battlefields where soldiers are at risk for concussions.

The second device is the BrainScope. It consists of a strip of material that covers six electrical wires. This strip is stuck to an athlete's forehead just like a large Band-Aid. It connects to an iPod-sized minicomputer that automatically collects a sample of the player's brainwaves. The computer then compares the player's brainwaves with a database of normal brainwaves collected from more than twenty thousand people by the device's inventor. This exam takes about ten minutes to complete.

Both DETECT and BrainScope are currently being tested by athletic teams and in emergency rooms to see if they really do what they are supposed to do. These devices may be available for commercial use in the near future if they prove to be useful in their clinical trials.

Myths and Facts

Loss of consciousness occurs in all people who have concussions.

Fact: ➡ Many years ago, being knocked out was considered the only sign and symptom of a concussion. Doctors now know that only about 10 percent of those who experience a concussion are knocked unconscious. Concussions that produce loss of consciousness are considered to be "serious" or Grade III concussions.

Concussions are less serious if they occur in children than in adults.

Fact: ➡ Young children who experience concussions heal more slowly and are at greater risk for long-term problems related to the concussion than adults. People's brains are not fully developed until they are in their early twenties. Concussions in childhood may keep parts of a child's brain from developing normally. Behavior and learning problems may occur in these children.

Male athletes are far more likely to get concussions than female athletes.

Fact: ➥ Overall, boys get concussions more frequently than girls because more boys participate in collision and contact sports than girls do. A study of high school soccer players conducted in 2007 showed that girls experienced 68 percent more concussions than boys. Experts believe that using smaller soccer balls in girls' games might eliminate some of these concussions. Girls are three times more likely to get concussions playing high school basketball than are boys.

three

WHAT ARE THE CONSEQUENCES OF CONCUSSIONS?

Sometime in your life, you may have a concussion and never even know about it. If you do experience a concussion, it's likely that your symptoms will disappear within a few hours. If you get a concussion while playing a sport, it will probably be mild. You may miss a practice or two but not miss a game. A few teens who have concussions, however, are not so lucky. They can develop problems, one of which is life-threatening and many of which are now thought to result in long-term trouble with memory and learning.

Post-Concussion Syndrome

Post-concussion syndrome can occur after any concussion. A syndrome is a group of signs and symptoms that occur together. Doctors use the combination of these signs

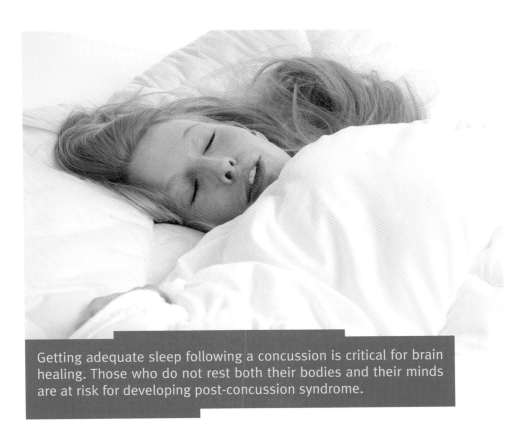

Getting adequate sleep following a concussion is critical for brain healing. Those who do not rest both their bodies and their minds are at risk for developing post-concussion syndrome.

and symptoms to identify a disease or condition. Some of the signs and symptoms of post-concussion syndrome include headache, dizziness, anxiety, problems with concentration, sleep irregularity, and personality changes. These are the very same symptoms that some people develop when they first experience a concussion. The problem is that the symptoms just don't go away. Post-concussion syndrome can last for months. But in most cases, symptoms disappear eventually. Experts now believe that people with concussions who don't adequately rest

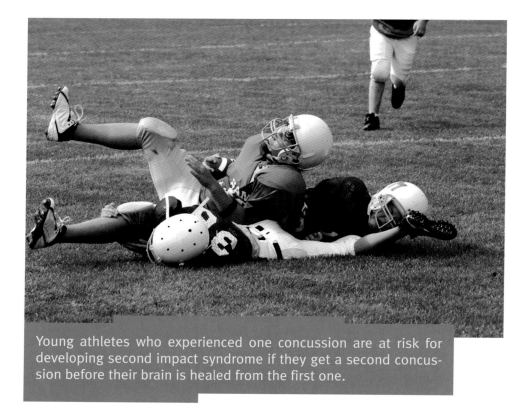

Young athletes who experienced one concussion are at risk for developing second impact syndrome if they get a second concussion before their brain is healed from the first one.

their bodies and their minds before returning to work or play are more likely to get post-concussion syndrome than those who do get adequate rest.

Second Impact Syndrome

Second impact syndrome is a rare, but potentially life-threatening, condition. It can occur if a person who has had a concussion is hit on the head and experiences a second concussion before his or her brain has healed from the first one. More than 50 percent of people who experience this die a short time after their second concussion. This syndrome is most likely to occur in young people. One reason is that many mild concussions are not witnessed or go undocumented in children and teens. It also takes longer for their brains to heal, so a second concussion may be deadly for them.

Second impact syndrome has never been seen in professional athletes, many of whom experience multiple concussions throughout their careers. There have been few proven cases in college athletes. Most of the cases that have occurred involved high school athletes. In several cases, the victim's coach was unaware that the athlete had experienced a previous head injury. Coaches are now much more diligent about informing an athlete's parents and other coaches when the athlete experiences a concussion. Hopefully, this action—and making sure that athletes are healed before they return to play—will eliminate second impact syndrome.

Learning Disabilities

Children who get concussions may have learning problems months or years later. Experts believe that as many as 5.3 million Americans suffer from mental or physical disabilities that are due to previous brain injuries. The Brain Injury Research Center at the Mount Sinai School of Medicine in New York City has done several studies looking at groups of children who've had head injuries. In one study, they worked with four hundred children in the New York school system who had problems learning. Almost 50 percent of these children had experienced a hard blow to the head before they developed their learning problems. Once the teachers learned of these children's head injuries, they changed the way they taught them. By giving them more time to solve problems and using techniques to help them concentrate, the teachers saw a great improvement in the children's ability to learn.

Punch-Drunk Syndrome

Boxing is a collision sport in which athletes intentionally hit each other. Although they wear helmets and mouthpieces to lessen the risk of getting concussions, almost all boxers are knocked out sooner or later, or at least suffer minor concussions. People who like boxing believe that boxers are no more likely than wrestlers or football players to get concussions. Others don't agree. They believe that boxing should be eliminated, especially as a sport for children and teens. At the present time, very few high schools have boxing teams, but there are boxing clubs that allow teens to participate.

The long-term effects of repeatedly suffering blows to the head can be seen in former boxers such as Muhammad Ali, one of the greatest heavyweight champions of all time. He has a type of Parkinson's disease (a progressive disease of the nervous system) called secondary parkinsonism, or post-traumatic parkinsonism, which has developed because of the repeated episodes of head trauma that he had while fighting. Like actor Michael J. Fox, who also has Parkinson's disease, Ali's muscles are very rigid. He has trouble talking, and he walks very slowly with an abnormal stride. These signs and symptoms are sometimes called punch-drunk syndrome because it's frequently seen in boxers. If the condition is accompanied by loss

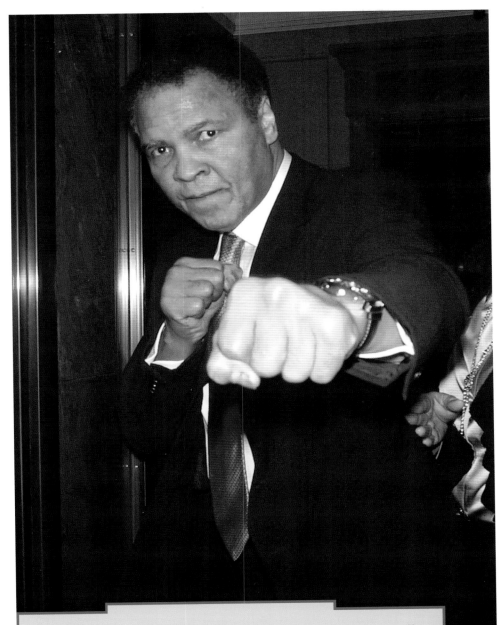

Muhammad Ali, pictured here in a visit to New York City, suffers from a form of Parkinson's disease caused by the many concussions he developed during his boxing career.

of memory, it may be called dementia pugilistica. The younger children or teens are when they begin to box, the more likely they are to receive concussions and the slower they are to heal. This is perhaps the best reason to suggest that boxing, if it's done at all, be only engaged in by adults whose brains are already fully developed.

Do the Benefits of Playing Sports Outweigh the Risks?

Participating in sports is fun and can improve your heath. Most athletes don't smoke, have less trouble maintaining an optimum weight, and tend to have more self-confidence. The friendships you make with your fellow athletes frequently last a lifetime. Good athletes may qualify for college athletic scholarships to help pay for tuition and other expenses. All of these positive aspects of sports participation have to be weighed against the risks of playing sports. The question is: how risky are the sports you like to play?

In 2006, 7.2 million high school students participated in organized sports in the United States. To try to determine how many injuries high school students got while playing sports, the Centers for Disease Control and Prevention (CDC) funded a study in which athletes from one hundred high schools took part. The study looked at the number and types of injuries these student athletes got when they participated in one or more of nine sports. These sports included football, soccer, basketball, baseball, and wrestling for boys, and soccer, basketball, softball, and volleyball for girls.

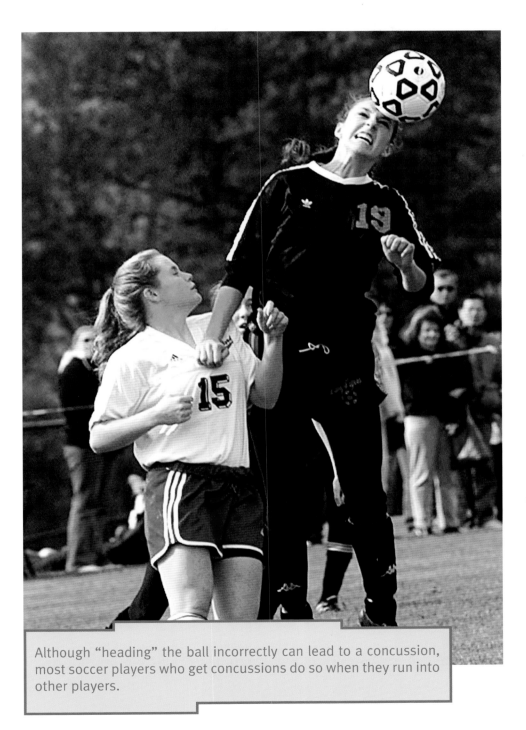

Although "heading" the ball incorrectly can lead to a concussion, most soccer players who get concussions do so when they run into other players.

The results of the study from the one hundred high schools were used to estimate the number of injuries among all U.S. high school students who participated in sports. It was estimated that 1.5 million injuries occurred among high school athletes playing one of the nine sports monitored in the 2005–2006 school year. Most were ankle injuries or muscle pulls, but about 136,000 (9 percent) of the injuries were concussions. The sport that boys liked the most, football, turned out to be the one in which most concussions occurred. This number was followed by girls' soccer, boys' soccer, and girls' basketball. Concussions occurred much less frequently in the other five sports.

The athletes in this study, with the exception of those playing baseball and softball, got most of their concussions when they ran into another player. This occurrence was true even in soccer, where "heading" the ball was once thought to be the most common cause of concussions in the sport. Football is the only collision sport in all the sports studies, so it isn't surprising that most of the concussions occurred in football players. The rest of the sports studied are considered to be contact sports where athletes may run into each other by accident but don't do it intentionally. Concussions are less likely to occur in these sports. As you may suspect, most concussions in baseball and softball occurred when players were hit with balls or bats.

Do Girls Get Concussions More Often Than Boys?

For many years, girls didn't participate in many team sports in high school or college. Now, they're active in almost every type of sport. As the number of girls participating in contact sports increases, so does the number of injuries they suffer. They appear to suffer more concussions than boys who play the same sports. A 2007 study of high school soccer players showed that girls experienced 68 percent more concussions than boys. In high school basketball, girls were three times more likely than boys to get concussions. Experts give several reasons why this is so. Girls have more flexible necks, and they have weaker neck and shoulder muscles to stabilize their heads. When girls get hit or "head" a ball, their heads have a tendency to rotate, rather than remain in a stable position. Rotational force is a common cause of concussions. Girls also have smaller ball-to-head ratios. So in heading a ball, their brains receive a greater impact from the ball than do those of boys. All these factors may contribute to the higher concussion rates in female soccer players compared with male soccer players.

Although several studies suggest that girls have more concussions than boys who play the same sport, it may be that boys have the same number or more concussions but just don't tell anyone about them. Many boys grow up believing that being macho and not admitting that they are hurt is a sign of manhood. Most girls, on the other hand, don't feel like they have to be as tough. It is all right for them to admit that they've been hurt.

As many boys as girls may get concussions. But the boys may elect to play while they are hurt and not report their injuries. Therefore, they may appear to get fewer concussions than girls do.

Chapter four

IS IT SAFE TO PARTICIPATE IN SPORTS IF I HAVE HAD A CONCUSSION?

"Is it safe to participate in sports if I have had a concussion?" If you had asked your doctor and your coach this question a few years ago, the answer would have been "Yes!" After reassuring you, they would have sent you right back into the game. Today, you might not get the same answer. Coaches and doctors now know it isn't always a good idea for athletes to return to play after having concussions. Each person who experiences one must be considered individually. A plan must be developed to determine if and when it is safe for the athlete to play again. Many factors are considered before making that decision. These include your age, if you've had a previous concussion, how severe your concussion was, if your neurocognitive tests showed abnormalities, and how quickly the abnormalities disappeared.

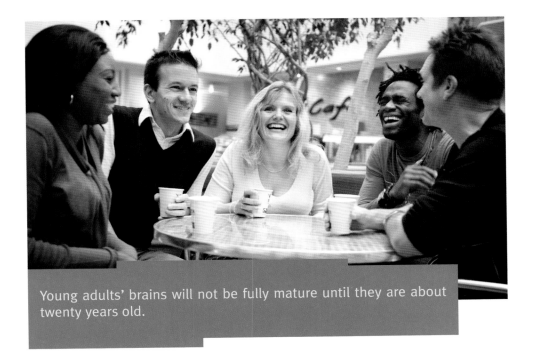

Young adults' brains will not be fully mature until they are about twenty years old.

What Does My Age Have to Do with It?

Not long ago, experts thought that children who had concussions were less likely to have problems than adults who had them. Now, just the opposite seems to be true. The brain is the last organ in the human body to mature. When humans are born, their brains are like computers that are waiting to be programmed. They have all the basic functions they need to stay alive, but they have a lot to learn before their brains are fully mature. Brain maturity is not reached until people are about twenty years old. The frontal lobes of the cerebral hemispheres are the last parts of the brain to fully mature. They are also the lobes that tend to be the most frequently injured in concussions. When children and teens experience severe concussions involving the frontal lobes, they may never develop the ability to plan for the future and may not be able to distinguish between right and wrong. As previously discussed, they may also have problems with learning and memory.

Multiple Concussions Can Lead to Big Problems

If you have a concussion, you are three times more likely to have a second concussion in the same sports season. After a second concussion, you are eight times more likely to have a third. Using neuropsychological testing, psychologists have shown that athletes who have experienced multiple concussions can't do as much mental work as they were able to do before. They get tired more easily, can't concentrate, and make many more mistakes. Michael W. Collins, a psychologist at the Sports Concussion Program at the University of Pittsburgh Medical Center, says that players who have suffered two or more concussions don't process information as fast as they did before their injuries or as fast as athletes who haven't had concussions. Collins compares these players to older, slower computers when he says, "They [players who suffer two or more concussions] were not processing information as quickly as those people who had one or zero concussions. It's kind of like your Pentium III computer becomes a Pentium II computer, or your 486 becomes a 386."

Grades of Concussions

Experts know that all concussions are not the same. Some are more serious than others and are more likely to cause long-term problems. Over the years, experts have used the signs and symptoms produced by concussions to develop more than forty different grading schemes to identify the seriousness of concussions. In most, Grade I concussions are the least serious, while Grade IV is the most serious. There are three grading schemes that are used most frequently. Each uses the signs and symptoms of confusion, amnesia, and loss of consciousness (LOC) to determine the severity of the concussion. An example of one of the three most widely used schemes is the Colorado Medical Society Concussion Grading Scheme:

- **Grade I Concussion (mild**) A concussion producing confusion, but no loss of consciousness.
- **Grade II Concussion (moderate)** A concussion producing confusion and post-traumatic amnesia (memory loss), but no loss of consciousness.
- **Grade III Concussion (serious)** A concussion that produces any loss of consciousness.

Grading schemes have become very important for evaluating athletes because they are used, along with the other factors mentioned above, to help determine when it is safe for an athlete to return to play.

Guidelines for Return to Play

"When can I play again?" is one of the questions you'll likely ask your coach if you experience a concussion. It isn't an easy question to answer because the answer depends on the grade of the concussion you experienced, how quickly your symptoms go away, and whether or not these symptoms return when you start a gradual, step-wise increase in your activity. It's likely that your school's athletic department has established a general plan for how to make the return-to-play decision for every athlete who gets a concussion. The general plan will be individualized to fit each player's situation. The goal, however, is always the same—to get you back to play as soon as it's safe for you to do so.

Coaches and team doctors frequently use the following guidelines, or variations of them, in making return-to-play decisions:

- You will likely not be allowed to return to play the same day you receive your concussion. Exceptions may be made to this rule if you are an older teen that has a very mild or Grade I concussion. If your confusion clears quickly and doesn't return as you do a few easy exercises on the sidelines, you may be allowed to return to play twenty to thirty minutes after your injury.
- You will be evaluated by your athletic trainer or team doctor shortly after your injury. That person may try to determine how severe your concussion is by using neurocognitive tests.

- You won't be left alone until your trainer or doctor decides that your symptoms are not getting worse.
- You will be asked to rest completely without doing any stressful physical or mental activity until all your symptoms are gone. It may be necessary for you to stay home from school and not attend social functions for at least twenty-four hours after your injury. This is the most important step in the entire process. It is very important that you rest your mind, as well as your body. Inadequate rest may make your recovery period much longer.
- When your symptoms are gone, you may be given a full set of neuropsychological tests to see if you have any impairment in your ability to think, solve problems, concentrate, or remember things.
- If these studies are normal, your athletic trainer or coach will start you on a step-wise return to activity over several days. If you remain symptom-free as you increase your activity, you will probably be able to return to your sport in seven to ten days.

Because you are young, your coach will be very cautious about letting you return to play too early. He or she knows that it takes longer for your brain to heal than it would for an older athlete. If you've had more than one concussion, your coach will be even more cautious. You may even be required to miss play for the rest of the season in order to be safe. If you have a third concussion, you may need to consider changing to a sport or other activity in which you are less likely to be hurt again.

Ten Great Questions to Ask a Doctor

1 Do concussions occur only if you get hit on the head?

2 What part of the brain is injured in a concussion?

3 Can you see these injuries on X-rays?

4 Do all people who have concussions get knocked out?

5 How long will it take the headache I got with my concussion to go away?

6 Why can't I remember what happened before I got hit on the head?

7 Do girls who play soccer and basketball get as many concussions as boys who play these sports?

8 When can I return to practice and competition after a concussion?

9 Does it make any difference how well my bicycle helmet fits as long as I wear it?

10 I've had two concussions this year. Should I consider giving up my contact sport?

five

HOW ARE CONCUSSIONS PREVENTED AND TREATED?

Prevention is the only treatment for concussions. Symptoms of concussions, such as headaches, can be treated with mild pain medications. But, otherwise, the brain must simply heal itself. Teens get most of their concussions while riding in or driving cars, in bicycle accidents, or while playing sports. The most important step you can take to decrease your risk of getting a concussion in a car wreck is to wear your seatbelt. If you make it a habit to put your seatbelt on every time you get in the car, you will soon do this automatically. If you're invited to ride with friends but the car is so crowded that there aren't enough seatbelts for everyone, don't accept the invitation. The most important action you can take to avoid getting a concussion while bicycling is to wear a bicycle helmet. It is illegal for kids under the age of sixteen to ride a bike without wearing a helmet in twenty-two states and the District of Columbia. Some U.S. states require all bicyclists to wear helmets. Fourteen states have no helmet laws. In fourteen others, local municipalities have helmet laws, but the states themselves do not. Many studies have shown that wearing a helmet reduces your risk of getting a concussion in a bicycle accident by about 85 percent. In spite of these results, it is estimated that fewer than 18 percent of all people wear bicycle helmets on a regular basis.

To find out why more young people didn't wear helmets, eight state chapters of the American Automobile Association (AAA), in conjunction with the Consumer Product Safety Commission, conducted a survey of 282 children between the ages of eight and thirteen. The first question the children were asked was, "What one thing would you change on bike helmets to get more kids to wear them?" Of those surveyed, 52 percent said they would change how the helmets looked. They wanted helmets to be "cool" so that they wouldn't look like geeks when wearing them. The second question the students were asked was, "What do you dislike about bike helmets?" Among respondents, 46 percent said they disliked them because they didn't fit. Students considered the chinstraps to be particularly uncomfortable and the helmets too heavy. Girls with ponytails also found them uncomfortable and wanted helmets designed for their hairstyle.

Helmet manufacturers and marketers took this survey to heart and began to make a variety of bicycle helmets to appeal to boys and girls of all ages. In 2007, about 25 percent of bicycle riders reported wearing helmets on a regular basis. Between 35

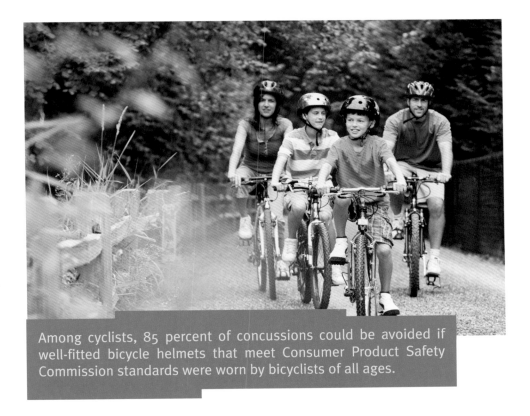

Among cyclists, 85 percent of concussions could be avoided if well-fitted bicycle helmets that meet Consumer Product Safety Commission standards were worn by bicyclists of all ages.

and 50 percent of people age sixteen or older reported wearing bicycle helmets regularly.

The helmet you wear when bicycling needs to be specifically constructed for bicycling and fit properly. It should also meet the standards set by the Consumer Product Safety Commission (see http://www.cpsc.gov). All helmets manufactured or sold in the United States must meet these standards. Look for a sticker inside the helmet that indicates the one you like has been approved. Before buying a helmet, make sure it fits properly and feels comfortable. The last step is to wear your helmet in the correct position, and make sure it's securely fastened.

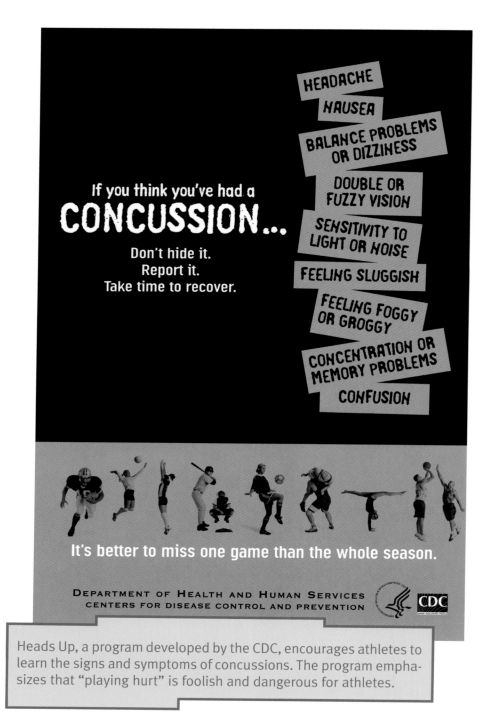

Heads Up, a program developed by the CDC, encourages athletes to learn the signs and symptoms of concussions. The program emphasizes that "playing hurt" is foolish and dangerous for athletes.

Many authorities recommend that bicycle helmets be worn when riding scooters, skating, or skateboarding. They can also be worn for ice skating and sledding. They should not, however, be worn while skiing or snowboarding. There are helmets specifically designed for these sports. They have outer shells that prevent anything from penetrating them, a middle shock-absorbing layer, and an inner insulating layer that keeps the skier's or snowboarder's head warm without additional headwear. The helmets also allow for goggle attachment. The Consumer Product Safety Commission estimates that each year, 11 skiing and snowboarding-related deaths and at least 7,700 head injuries (2,600 in children) could be prevented or reduced in severity if everyone wore helmets.

Efforts to decrease the number of concussions experienced by athletes participating in sports are being concentrated in three areas: improving education about concussions, improving equipment to protect athletes, and improving and enforcing the rules of play in each sport.

Why Is Education Important in Preventing Concussions?

For many years, concussions were not considered to be very important, so little effort was made to tell people about them. Since scientists have discovered how many problems can be caused by concussions, however, they've been promoting programs to bring concussions to the attention of coaches, athletic trainers, and especially athletes and their parents. The CDC is leading this educational effort with Heads Up, a program created for high school athletes, their parents, and their coaches.

The CDC has developed packets of information that are available free of charge either online or by mail. Among the items in the packets are fact sheets for athletes and their parents. There is also a guide for coaches that specifically deals with concussions in high school athletes. The fact sheets and coach's guide give basic information about concussions, including signs and symptoms to look out for. The fact sheet for athletes emphasizes how important it is for you to tell your coach if you think you've had a concussion. Playing with a concussion is not macho or smart. Another point made in the fact sheet is that resting your body and mind until your brain heals after a concussion is crucial. As the fact sheet says, "It is better to miss one game than the whole season."

This program and others give you information about concussions. But learning how to play your sport correctly is also necessary to help prevent concussions. Two moves that coaches teach to help protect their athletes are keeping the head up when making a tackle in football and heading a ball correctly in soccer. Those who learn these lessons and others pertaining to their particular sport and apply them every time they play will have far fewer concussions than those who don't practice what they're taught.

Super Helmets and New Protective Equipment Help Prevent Concussions

Several football helmets have been, and are being, developed that can give coaches, trainers, and doctors information about what is happening to the brains of their players. At least three university football teams are testing football helmets that are equipped with accelerometers. Accelerometers are springlike devices that are placed between the protective cushions inside of helmets. When a player's helmet is hit, these devices measure the force of the blow to the helmet and, therefore, to the head of its wearer. This information is wirelessly sent from a transmitter in the helmet to a small computer on the sidelines. Every player who is wearing one of these helmets can be followed throughout the game with each impact to his head being recorded. Team physicians and trainers who monitor players can determine how much force is being applied to an athlete's brain and if it's great enough to cause a concussion. If the force of a particular blow is great enough, team physicians and trainers carefully watch the athlete that experienced the blow to make sure he or she doesn't develop signs of a concussion.

Information gained from studies employing these special helmets is being used not only to monitor players while they play but also to improve helmet designs. By increasing protective padding in helmets in areas where most impacts occur, the helmets give added protection. Other advances in helmet design improve the fit of helmets. A study conducted in high school athletic programs showed that only about 15 percent of football helmets fit properly and that coaches spend a lot of time trying to find helmets that fit their players. If helmets don't fit properly, they can't provide maximum protection.

Other equipment changes that may make sports safer include softer baseballs and soccer balls. Baseballs and softballs are now

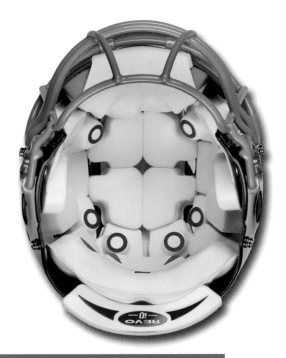

Some teams use football helmets that contain sensors to measure the severity and location of head impacts. Information gained from these sensors helps to monitor athletes for concussions.

being constructed with softer, spongier inner cores. If these balls are adopted for official play, it is hoped that their use will result in fewer head and facial injuries in players hit by balls. Some helmets used in baseball are now being fitted with facemasks. These will help protect players from facial injuries and may also decrease the number of concussions experienced by baseball players.

Although most concussions in soccer are experienced when players run into each other, some occur when players head a ball. This is especially true with girls, since their neck and shoulder muscles are not as bulky or strong as those of boys. Soccer officials are now considering the wisdom of using smaller and lighter balls in women's soccer to prevent some of these injuries. At the present time, the size and weight of soccer balls used in a particular match are determined by the age of the players. It doesn't take into consideration the structural differences between girls and boys. The use of helmets in soccer has also been considered, and helmets have been developed for the special needs of soccer players. However, these have not been widely accepted or used by soccer teams or organizations.

Enforcing Rules of Play Is Important in Preventing Concussions

Most sports rules were developed for specific reasons. Some make the game more interesting and fun to play. Many, however, were adopted to make games safer. Rule changes were made in football, for instance, that prohibit spearing (using the helmet to block or punish an opponent) and using the face-mask to tackle an opponent. If these rules are enforced, they make the game much safer for everyone. In educating their athletes, coaches emphasize that athletes hurt themselves and others when they fail to follow the rules of the game. Game officials must also be educated in the importance of enforcing the rules of play. Well-officiated games are critical in preventing concussions.

What Can You Do?

Ten steps you should take to avoid a concussion and prevent them in others are the following:

1. Always wear your seatbelt when riding in a car.
2. Get a good helmet that is appropriate to the sport or activity you are participating in, and wear it correctly every time you play.
3. Get in shape before starting a new sport or recreational activity.
4. Learn the correct way to perform the various skills of your sport.
5. Always follow the rules of the game.
6. Learn the signs and symptoms of concussions, and teach them to your friends and parents. The more people who know them, the better.
7. If you think you may have experienced a concussion, don't stay in the game. Tell your coach or trainer so that you can be properly evaluated.
8. Keep an eye on your teammates to make sure they don't develop signs of concussions. Report them to your coach if they do.
9. Teach your younger siblings how important it is to wear their helmets every time they bike or skate. Show them how to wear them properly because helmets won't do much good if they're too loose or are in the wrong position.

10. Get together with your friends and sponsor a concussion awareness booth at a school or sporting event. You'll be able to get help for this activity from many adults, and you'll have the satisfaction of knowing that you're sharing information with others that can prevent them from having problems in the future.

Concussions are one of the most serious medical problems at the high school level. When parents, coaches, trainers, doctors, officials, and athletes work together for a common cause such as preventing concussions, the likelihood of success is high. You and your teammates are the ones who will benefit from this effort.

abnormal Unusual or unexpected, especially in a way that causes alarm or anxiety.

axon A long, stringlike structure in the neurons of the brain that carries messages in the form of electrical impulses from cell bodies to other parts of the brain.

baseline A place from which to start; a test with which to compare another test.

clinical trial A research study used to evaluate the effectiveness and safety of medications or medical devices by monitoring their effects on a large number of people.

cognitive Involving cognition, which is the process of knowing and being aware—thinking, learning, and judging.

computed tomography (CT) A computerized method of taking a special picture of the brain in which the brain is seen in cross-sectional slices.

concentrate The ability to focus on or pay attention to something.

consciousness Mentally awake and alert.

consequence An event or action that occurs because of something that happened before.

coordination The ability of various parts of the body to work together to make a task possible.

hemisphere One half of a rounded structure, such as the cerebrum of the brain.

impairment The loss of part or all of a physical or mental ability, such as the ability to see, walk, or learn.

magnetic resonance imaging (MRI) A method of taking a picture of the brain that involves using powerful magnets and radio waves to look at the brain's structure.

neuron A nerve cell, usually consisting of a cell body, axon, and dendrites, that transmits nerve impulses and is the basic functional unit of the nervous system.

nutrient Nourishment or food.

orientation Knowledge of who you are, where you are, and what time it is.

psychologist A professional who is trained in the study of the mind, including cognitive functions and behavior.

stimulate To cause physical activity in something such as a nerve or cell.

traumatic Of or relating to a physical injury or wound to the body.

vacant Empty or blank.

American Brain Coalition
6257 Quantico Lane North
Maple Grove, MN 55331
(763) 557-2913
Web site: http://www.americanbraincoalition.org
  This nonprofit organization seeks to advance the understanding of the functions of the brain and reduce the
  burden of brain disorders through advocacy.

Brain Injury Association of America
1608 Spring Hill Road, Suite 110
Vienna, VA 22182
(703) 761-0750
Web site: http://www.biausa.org
  Founded in 1980, this national organization and its
  forty chartered state affiliates provide information,
  education, and support to assist 3.2 million Americans
  currently living with brain injuries.

Brain Injury Resource Center
P.O. 84151
Seattle, WA 98124-5451
(206) 621-8558
Web site: http://www.headinjury.com

This agency offers factual information on brain injuries and rehabilitation from them. It maintains the Head Injury Hotline, at (206) 621-8558.

Brain Trauma Foundation
523 East 72nd Street, 8th Floor
New York, NY 10021
(212) 722-0608
Web site: http://www.braintrauma.org
   The goal of this organization is to improve the outcome of TBI patients by developing best practice guidelines, conducting clinical research, and educating medical personnel.

Centers for Disease Control and Prevention
1600 Clifton Road
Atlanta, GA 30333
(800) 232-4636
Web site: http://www.cdc.gov
   This federal government agency provides information about health-related problems. Its Heads Up program educates athletes, parents, and coaches about concussions.

National Brain Injury Research, Treatment, and Training
   Foundation
P.O. Box 528
Huntersville, NC 28070
(704) 992-1424
Web site: http://www.nbirtt.org

This organization provides support for research, treatment, and training in brain injury through research grants, contracts, and small business grants.

National Institute of Neurological Disorders and Stroke
NIH Neurological Institute
P.O. Box 5801
Bethesda, MD 20824
(301) 496-5751
Web site: http://www.ninds.nih.gov
    The mission of this federal government agency is to reduce the burden of neurological disease—a burden borne by every age group and segment of society worldwide.

National Youth Sports Safety Foundation
One Beacon Street, Suite 3333
Boston, MA 02108
(617) 367-6677
Web site: http://www.nyssf.org
    This is an educational organization dedicated to reducing the number and severity of injuries sustained by youth in sports and fitness programs.

Safe Kids Canada
180 Dundas Street W, Suite 2105
Toronto, ON M5G 128
Canada
(416) 813-7288
Web site: http://www.safekidscanada.ca

The Canadian branch of this international organization pro-
motes effective strategies to prevent unintentional injuries to
children.

Think First Foundation of Canada
750 Dundas Street W, Suite 3-314
Toronto, ON M6J 353
Canada
(416) 915-6565
Web site: http://www.thinkfirst.ca
   This Canadian national nonprofit organization is dedicated
   to the prevention of brain and spinal cord injuries through
   education.

Web Sites

Due to the changing nature of Internet links, Rosen Publishing
has developed an online list of Web sites related to the subject
of this book. This site is updated regularly. Please use this link
to access this list:

http://www.rosenlinks.com/faq/conc

Boesky, Lisa. *When to Worry: How to Tell If Your Teen Needs Help—and What to Do About It*. New York, NY: AMACOM, 2007.

Brynie, Faith Hickman. *101 Questions Your Brain Has Asked About Itself But Couldn't Answer Until Now*. Rev. ed. Minneapolis, MN: Twenty-First Century, 2008.

Carson, Dale. *The Teen Brain Book: Who and What Are You?* Madison, CT: Bick Publishing House, 2004.

Hains, Bryan C. *Brain Disorders* (Gray Matter). New York, NY: Chelsea House Publishers, 2005.

Hossler, Phil, and Ron Savage. *Getting A-Head of Concussion*. Wake Forest, NC: Lash and Associates Publishing, 2006.

Hughes, Pat. *Open Ice*. New York, NY: Windy Lamb Books, 2005.

Mason, Douglas. *The Mild Traumatic Brain Injury Workbook: Your Program for Regaining Cognitive Function and Overcoming Emotional Pain*. Oakland, CA: New Harbinger Publications, 2004.

McCrea, Michael. *Mild Traumatic Brain Injury and Post Concussion Syndrome: The New Evidence Base for Diagnosis and Treatment*. New York, NY: Oxford University Press, 2008.

Nowinski, Chris. *Head Games: Football's Concussion Crisis from the NFL to Youth Leagues*. Plymouth, MA: Drummond Publishing Group, 2006.

Pearson, Mary. *Adoration of Jenna Fox*. New York, NY: Henry Holt and Company, 2008.

Phillips, Sherre Florence. *The Teen Brain*. New York, NY: Chelsea House Publishers, 2007.

Solomon, Gary, Karen Johnston, and Mark Lovell. *The Heads-Up on Sport Concussion*. Champaign, IL: Human Kinetics Publishers, 2005.

Zevin, Gabriella. *Memoirs of a Teenage Amnesiac*. New York, NY: Farrar, Straus and Giroux, 2007.

index

About the Author

Linda Bickerstaff is a retired surgeon who's had personal experience with concussion while playing softball in high school. She has written several magazine articles for teens on health topics. She has also written several books for teens, including *Technology and Infertility: Assisted Reproduction and Modern Society* (Science and Society) and *Cocaine: Coke and the War on Drugs* (Drug Abuse and Society).

Photo Credits

Cover, p. 5 © www.istockphoto.com; p. 7 © Nucleus Medical Art/Visuals Unlimited; p. 8 © www.istockphoto.com/David Freund; p. 10 © Don W. Fawcett/Photo Researchers; p. 14 © www.istockphoto.com/Chris Price; p. 17 © Richard T. Nowitz/ Photo Researchers; p. 19 © Courtesy of UPMC Sports Medicine Concussion Program; p. 22 © Dr. Michelle Laplaca/Georgia Institute of Technology/Emory University; p. 27 © www. istockphoto.com/Andreas Reh; p. 28 © www.istockphoto.com/ James Boulette; p. 31 © Arnoldo Magnani/Getty Images; p. 33 © Tony Savino/The Image Works; p. 37 © www.istockphoto.com/ Chris Schmidtt; p. 45 © Andersen Ross/Getty Images; p. 46 CDC; p. 50 © Courtesy of Riddell.

Designer: Nicole Russo; Editor: Kathy Kuhtz Campbell; Photo Researcher: Marty Levick